CW01471652

Wicca Spells

Practical Wicca Candle Charms for Beginners: How to use crystals, candles, runes, herbs and moon magic to cast powerful spells and master secrets and rituals

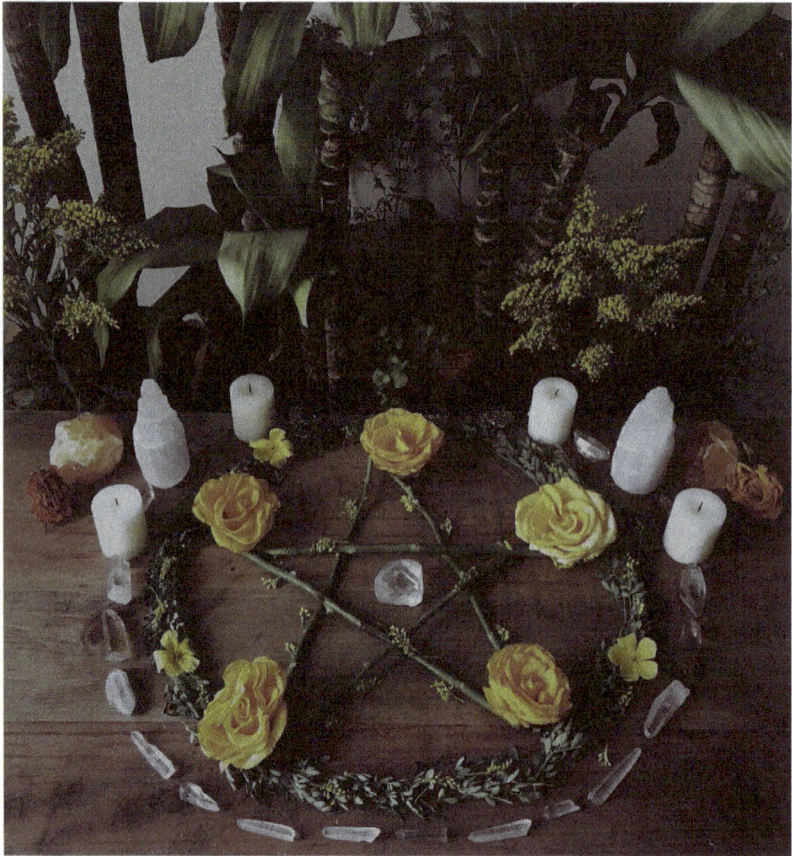

Table of Contents

Introduction

Congratulations on buying *Wicca Spells* and thank you for doing so. Wicca is considered as one of the fastest growing religions in the United States and in the Western World. Unlike what was previously believed, Wicca promotes harmony and peace. By reading the following chapters of this book, you will know the origin and history of Wicca, Wiccan beliefs, rituals, and ethics, and the eight Wiccan sabbaths as well as the esbats—rituals devoted to the moon and the divine triple goddess. This book will also cover what it means to worship the god and goddess, and what they represent in their various aspects. A thorough introduction to the Wheel of the Year, the meaning of the days of the week, and a full spellbook for both the beginner and expert practitioner of magic is included. The spells in this book include chantings, rituals, and what you need to perform these spells can be commonly found in the household. The spells in this book are so simple that even the beginner can easily follow them. Spells for wealth, abundance, luck in money and business, self-awareness, self-empowerment, love, romance, being open in receiving love in one's life, invisibility, protection of the home, protection of one's self or vehicle, and safe travels are just some of the spells included in *Wicca Spells*.

Wicca Spells will ready you as you take a journey of a lifetime. You already did the first step by purchasing this book. Now all you have to do is take the second step and learn the spells.

There are plenty of books on this subject on the market, thanks again for choosing this one! Every effort was made to ensure it is full of as much useful information as possible, please enjoy!

The Time of the Waning Moon

The waning moon is a time of reduction, of things moving away, and winding down. It can be a good time for reflection for hard work when obstacles no longer slow us down. It is a good time for magical work involving getting rid of bad luck or illness as well as reducing something that's run rampant or gone unchecked for too long such as one's appetite, party habits, unrequited desire for another person, procrastination, weight gain, fatigue, or being the object of gossip. Instead of looking at the waning moon as a time of loss, use it to your advantage. We are not meant to be in a constant state of reception and acquisition—sometimes, we need to be able to let go, shed our skins, discard that which no longer serves us. Just as the lushness of Summer dies down in Autumn and is absorbed back into the Earth at Winter so we, too, need to reduce and recycle some things in our lives that have reached their peak. It is healthy to be able to take stock of one's life and recognize aspects whose time has come and gone.

Magic involving protection, breaking bad habits, weight loss, eating healthier, getting an advantage over addictions, removing negativity, rising above one's enemies, and even monetary gain can be performed during a waning moon. Sometimes we get stuck in a rut and cannot see the opportunities in front of us. If you're feeling courageous and desire great, successful change,and perform a spell for an exciting new career during a waning moon.

The Dark Moon

The dark moon's energy can be unsettling for some. Like the full moon, the dark moon is a mirror of the self, though it shows us our shadow side rather than the side the world sees day to day. A concept of a shadow self in Wiccan and other pagan faiths is that we all have darker leanings, habits, responses, or traits that we may not be proud of, or even ashamed of. However, the god and goddess support us as being our authentic selves as humans. They teach us that being human is nothing to be ashamed of.

Sometimes our shadows, when properly understood, accepted, and controlled, can be some of our strongest features. Doing shadow work under a dark moon is a way to courageously explore one's self, and come to terms with it, thus emerging stronger, happier, and more complete.

Magic to be performed on a dark moon may involve protection, invisibility, drawing the truth out from obscurity, raising self-confidence, accepting one's shadow traits, forgiveness of one's self or of another, making a pact to strive for something, and banishing negative energy from one's person, life, or home.

Blue Moons and Blood Moons

A blue moon is a second full moon in a month and presents a wonderful opportunity to perform magic that focuses on good fortune and luck. The blue moon increases the full moon's potency even more so nearly any magic focusing on positivity and gain should be performed at this time.

A blood moon is the result of something called a *syzygy* where the Earth, Sun, and Moon are almost exactly in line with each other. As the Earth moves between the other two heavenly bodies, its shadow appears on the Moon. This shadow is called an *umbra*.

A blood moon is when a level 5 red eclipse occurs. The illusion of the red color is caused by the Earth's shadow and presents an interesting time to perform magical spells. As the blood moon is the result of the Sun, Moon, and Earth joining forces, so to speak, so we can focus on spells that address our outer selves, inner knowledge and intuition, and how we are grounded in knowledge and experience. Breakthrough spells for career, a new book deal, meeting the lover of your dreams, overcoming a physical impairment, or any epiphany regarding self-awareness can be cast during a blood moon. Who knows—you might just win the lottery!

Chapter 1 Spells

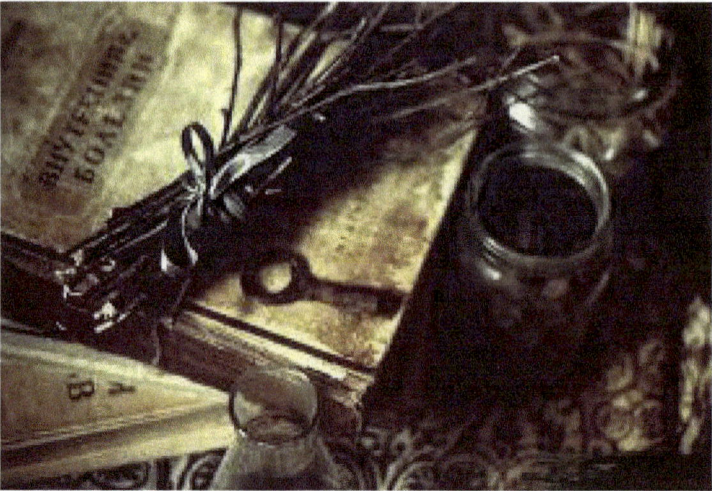

Preparing To Work With Magic

There are many things to consider when you decide to cast a spell. The time of day, for instance, as well the current moon phase, day of the week, and what natural items are available during that season.

When you're first getting started working with magic, preparation is advised so you have a clear plan of strategy. As you become more experienced, you'll find that you're more comfortable with "winging it" since you'll have committed to memory some of the things you've worked with in the past.

The number one question to ask yourself before you cast a spell is what do you desire to make happen, to change?

Never Ask "How"

Your own attitude is perhaps the most powerful ingredient in any magic spell. It's human nature to seek the "how" and the "why" of things but when it comes to witchcraft and Wiccan magic, the only answers to how and why must be *because the universe will hear me and make it so* and *because I will it to be*. That's it. You are one being in a universe of energy. Trust in the fabric of things to fetch you the result you called for and let the questions leave your mind as you trust in your own ability to perform magic.

Timing Your Spell

If there is a great need to cast a spell and time is of the essence, then by all means, cast it when you must. If you have the luxury of time, however, this is a guideline as to when to plan to do the work:

Lunar Phases

- **Waxing Moon:** Abundance, looking for a new job, looking for a new home, success with healing from an injury or illness*, new love, strengthening a relationship or family bond, spells to help a garden or plant grow, blessings for babies or young animals. *A healing spell during a waxing moon will focus on increasing the immune system, strength, or vitality of the person rather than focusing on the illness or injury itself.

- **Full Moon:** The most auspicious time to perform abundance spells, self-empowerment, spells for passion, success, beauty, spells for good luck in finance and business, blessings to consecrate tools, magic items, magic sachets or amulets, jewelry, crystals, potions, and elixirs.

- **Waning Moon:** banishing spells, spells to reduce the impact or influence of something, spells to cleanse a space or person of negativity, spells for help with healing from an illness or injury*, spells to reduce anxiety, worry, or depression. Spells to make things smaller and less significant. *A healing spell during a waning moon will focus on reducing the impact of the injury or lessening the infection or sickness in the person.

- **New Moon:** Spells for change within one's self, a new start, getting rid of bad habits and replacing them with good habits, spells to discern the truth of a matter, spells for commitment to a long-term goal.

- **Dark Moon:** Spells for protection, stealth, and invisibility. Spells for justice. Spells to honor the ancestors.

Days of the Week

- **Monday:** Spells that honor the moon or the divine feminine, spells for new beginnings. The moon's energy is full of mystery and it is the opposite of the bold, forward sun. This day is best for introspection and self-discovery rather than any spell that requires action. This is a good day for water magic, and the water element is strong on this day.

- **Tuesday:** This is a good day for spellwork involving self-empowerment and rising above or besting one's enemies. It is ruled by the god of war, Mars, and so avoid using bright red or any peppery spice such as cinnamon to ensure your magic isn't too incendiary. This is a good day to charge talismans and items of protection.

- **Wednesday:** Wear an item of red on this day for good luck. Wednesday is sacred to Mercury, god of communication. A good day for magic involving contracts, good news, good luck, and partnerships. A good time to do spellwork for financial success and success in business as well as safe travel and messages or work well-received.

- **Thursday:** This day is ideal for luck and good fortune spells as well as spells for abundance, money magic, and spells for good healthy. This day is ruled by Jupiter, god of luck. Also a good day for work involving justice and to gain favor with authorities. A good time for blessings of the home or vehicles.

- **Friday:** Friday is ruled by Venus but it is also sacred to other goddesses such as the Yoruban goddess of unbridled passion, the marketplace, lightning, and the graveyard. It is a heady day filled with possibility. A good day for love and attraction magic, success in attracting clients and customers, attracting the attention of someone you desire, and spells for beauty and self-confidence.

- **Saturday:** Ruled by Saturn, this day is best for protection magic, getting in touch with the beloved dead, creating wards of protection for person, home, and property. It is a good day for divination.

- **Sunday:** This day is, of course, ruled by the Sun. It is a day well-suited for spells for good health and vitality, successful planting, luck in money, and magic involving career and business.

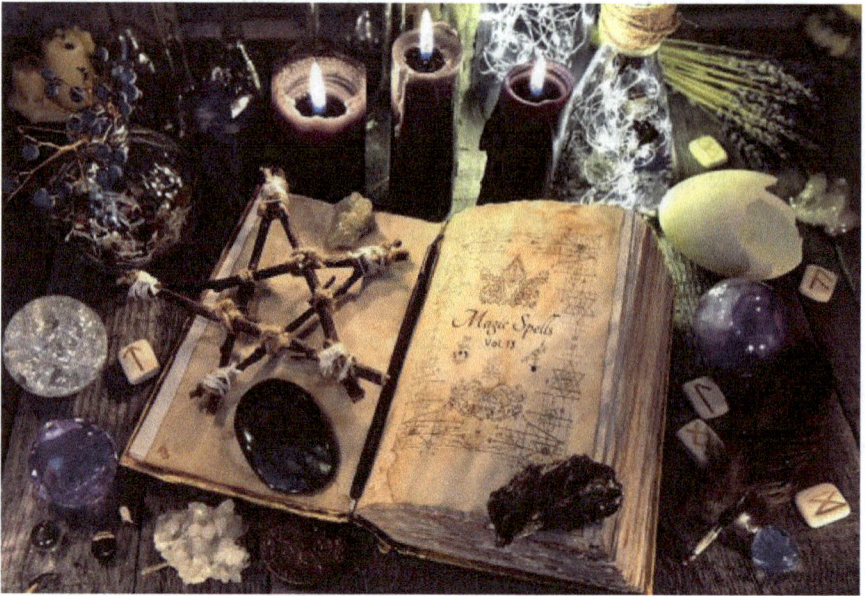

Understanding Your Intent

One of the most essential parts of witchcraft is having a clearly defined goal and intent before you begin. Take some time to write down what you wish to accomplish with the spell. The more specific, the better. It can be a series of results, step by step. Study your intention and determine if it's truly the right time to cast this spell.

> **A note about casting spells on other people:** This is a subject often hotly debated in pagan circles. In Wicca, there is an explicit rule that you should not cast a spell on someone without their permission. If that person is in need of healing, encouragement, or better luck, a well-intentioned spell cast on their behalf is a good thought, but without their consent, it is a violation of their energy and their rights.

Additionally, spells to make someone "fall in love" or become attracted to you or another person are also against Wiccan values. They're also just a very bad idea. Bending the will of another person is nearly impossible through magic. The will of a human being is one of the strongest forces on Earth. The most common scenario that occurs as the result of a powerful love spell is an obsession—an unhealthy attachment to the person who cast the spell. This is not true love and it will not end well: obsession leads to codependency, or at worst, revulsion. The best way to attract true love is to focus on being the happiest, healthiest, most self-respecting, radiant person you can be, as well as being open to attracting love.

When you're in need to protect yourself or someone else from a specific person, casting a spell to create a protective barrier is permissible. Guarding yourself from negativity or ill will is not against Wiccan ethics, nor is a spell of return: casting a spell that returns any negative energy to the person who sent it.

Preparing Yourself and Your Space

Before you get ready to cast your spell, take some time to cleanse yourself and your workspace. If you need a shower, have one—*then* spiritually cleanse yourself. It is said you "have to get rid of the worldly dirt before you tackle the spiritual dirt". Spiritual cleansing can be achieved by using sage, palo santo wood, rosemary, Florida water, or holy water (which you can make at home using nature-collected water such as river or rain water, and adding salt. Saltwater is also good for this). If smudging (using a smoking herb bundle like sage or rosemary), move the bundle counterclockwise (called widdershins in Wiccan ceremony) over the areas of your body, head to foot.

After you've cleansed yourself, do the same for your sacred space.

Having the Proper Presence of Mind

When you're ready to cast your circle, take a few moments to ease your mind into a relaxed state. You may sit before your altar or workspace, keeping your posture straight, and breathing deeply, through your stomach. Empty your mind of thoughts. Just drift for a while, relax yourself into the best state of mind for magical work.

Casting a Circle

Before you begin your magical work, it's important to enclose the space you're working *in*. The reasoning behind this is that you're about to use your own energy to cast a spell. There will be a point of focus, of some sort, that your energy will be aimed upon. A circle makes it easier to keep your energy in a small, focused area. Additionally, a protective circle will keep out any unknown, unseen, energies that might interfere with your work.

You should have a good idea where the four directions are in relation to your workspace or altar. Ideally, your altar should face North but if that's not possible don't worry. Another solution is to have a portable altar that you place in the center of your room when it's time for spellcasting. A wooden footstool or small coffee table works well for this.

Two easy ways to determine the directions if you don't have a compass: look up your home on Google Maps or Google Earth or download a compass app for your phone.

When you're ready to cast your circle, stand, and holding your wand or athame, point to the North.

By the North where she dwells in power, by the East where she sings her song, by the South where the fires of her passion ignite, by the West where her waters run deep.

You can add a verse for the god as well, if you like:

By the North where he guards his fortress, by the East where he sails for home, by the South where he lights his fiery torch, by the West where he quenches his thirst.

Then say:

The circle is cast.

Whenever you are finished with a spell, the last step will always be to recite the Casting Words:

By the power of three times three, I cast this spell so humbly, to harm no one, nor to bring harm to me, I cast this spell – SO MOTE IT BE.

When your work is done, you can open the circle by reciting the same words that you used to cast it, then instead of saying "the circle is cast", say "the circle is open, but unbroken."

Grounding

One of the most important steps in magical work is called grounding. Your circle will contain an enormous amount of energy, and this energy will linger even after you've opened the circle. It can cause sleeplessness, nervousness, and restlessness in the spellcaster. It's essential that you *ground* this energy so it doesn't disturb the rest of your day or night.

You can accomplish grounding in a few different ways: you can kneel on the floor of your workspace, palms down, and feel the energy flow through you, into the floor, down to the Earth. Picture the room draining of the magical energy the way a bathtub drains water.

A second approach is to go outside, barefoot, and stand on land or rock for several minutes. Picture the energy draining out of you, down into the Earth.

Candle Magic

Using a candle for a spell's focus is one the most simple and effective spells you can cast. Choose a color to enhance the focus, depending on what type of spell you're looking for. Additionally, when making a charm bag or amulet, consult the color guide when choosing the color of your material.

white: for a clear, focused mind, to purify, to cleanse, a neutral candle for any magic except banishing and protection.

blue: healing, obtaining wisdom, a peaceful home, patience.

purple: use for divination magic, prophetic dreams, creating peace between two people or groups, connection to the god and goddess, connection to the spirit world.

red: passion, strength, courage, robust health.

orange: success, good fortune, wealth, attraction, vitality.

yellow: sensuality, friendship, happiness, money magic, communication.

black: protection, transformation, connection with ancestors, enlightenment, potential.

brown: a happy home, prosperity, creativity, fertility, stamina, good investment of wealth and energy, spells for animals.

pink: magic for children and babies, angelic healing, spirituality, affection.

gold: financial success, divination, past life memory.

silver: wisdom, luck in love, invisibility, protection from negativity, psychic power.

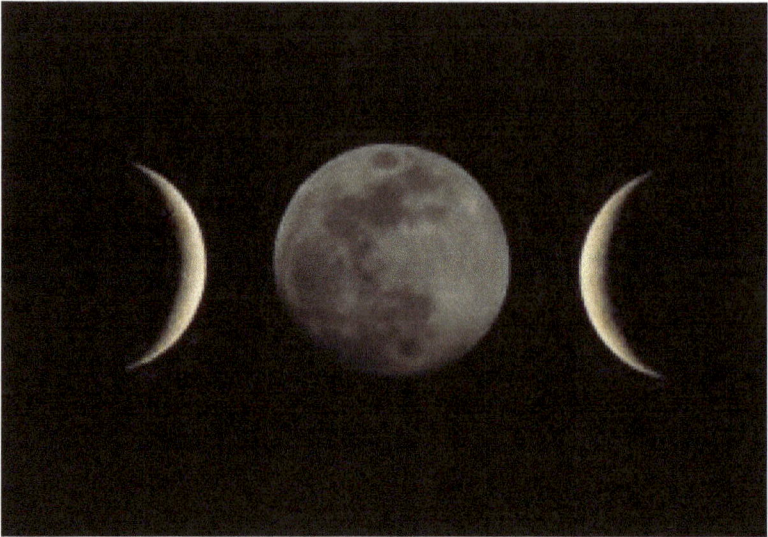

Spells For Personal Empowerment

Earth and Sky Spell

What you'll need:

- bay leaf

- basil

- lemon balm

- a small rock of obsidian

- a small rock of tiger's eye

- a small cloth pouch (or you can sew your own if the latter then include needle, thread, and scissors in the items before you cast the circle)

- white tealight or short taper candle

  Do this spell at night. Cast your circle, then raise your arms up, fingertips towards the ceiling. Feel the energy of the night sky, all its planets, moons, and stars, channeling down into your circle, swirling around until your circle fills with energy like water fills a glass. When your circle is full, imagine the energy glowing bright white, then allow your arms to drop comfortably at your sides.

Light the candle. Place the bay leaf in the pouch and say, "Tonight I give myself the gift of strength, and of endurance."

Place the basil in the pouch and say, "Tonight I give myself the gift of wealth, and of the courage to conquer my fears."

Place the lemon balm in the pouch and say, "Tonight I give myself the gift of love, and of success."

Place the obsidian in the pouch and say, "Tonight I give myself the gift of protection from negativity."

Place the tiger's eye in the pouch and say, "Tonight I give myself the gift of clarity, and of integrity."

Tie the pouch, or sew it closed if it's handmade. Hold the pouch in your hands and slowly move it clockwise (called "sunwise" in Wicca), above the candle. (Don't burn your hands).

Say: "Tonight I cast this spell for me, to reach for the stars and cast my net to the sea, to walk the Earth in discovery, to live my life happily."

Focus on the bag of charms, and imagine yourself in scenarios where you are happy, successful, and powerful. When you are ready, recite the Casting Words.

Inner Power Candle Spell

What you'll need:

- a white, brown, or blue taper candle

- a mixture of clove, juniper, and rose oils to anoint the candle. Handle the clove oil with care—only one or two drops of each are needed.

- a small, thin, paintbrush.

- a small dish on which to burn the candle.

- pink or kosher salt.

- matches to light the candle—preferable over a lighter, as metal should not strike a holy flame, but in a pinch, use what's available.

Cast your circle and draw the energy down from the universe. With the paintbrush, anoint the candle in the oil mixture, using brushstrokes that move from the back of the candle towards the front, and you. Work from the base of the candle towards the wick. Imagine yourself in moments of great personal power.

Light the candle and say:

"As it burns, so I learn. As it dances, so I turn. As it flickers, so I grow. As it melts, so my troubles go."

Move your hands above the candle as if you were drawing the healing energy of the flame towards you. Do this as you repeat:

"Flame of power, imbue me with your strength."

Sit in quiet contemplation for as long as your comfortable, imagining yourself overcoming obstacles, and obtaining happiness, and a peaceful heart. When you're ready, open the circle and allow the candle to burn down. After the candle is burned you can dispose of the wax and salt either by tossing them in a crossroads, or by burying them.

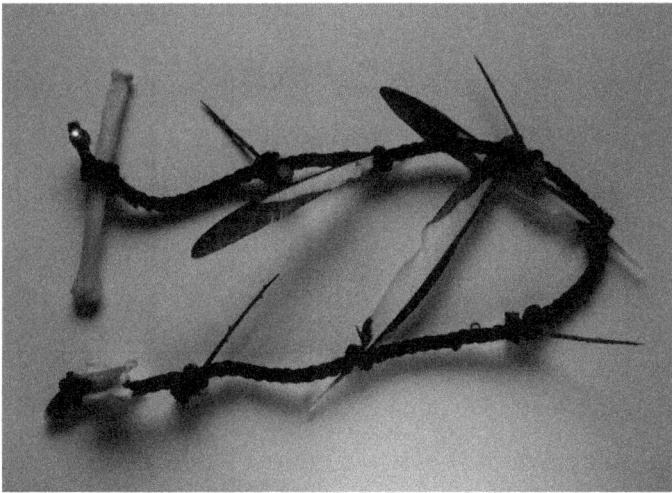

Spell to Nourish the Heart

What you'll need:

- pink quartz

- rose petals

- lemon balm

- lemon essential oil

Do this spell on a new, waxing, or full moon.

Cast your circle in the bathroom. Fill a bath and add five drops of the lemon essential oil to it. Add the rose petals and lemon balm. After you've gotten into the bath, add the pink quartz. As you sit in the bath, close your eyes and imagine a pink, healing light gleaming on the water. Imagine your body soaking up this healing energy. Feel your heart glowing with happiness and warmth that radiates throughout your entire body.

When you are ready, repeat these words:

"I am worthy of love, and I am capable of love.

I am worthy of peace, and I am capable of peace.

I am worthy of happiness, and I am capable of happiness.

All good things are possible. May they come into my life as blessings."

When you're finished with the bath, allow the water to drain and pat yourself dry (do not rub or wipe) with a towel from your feet up to your head. Discard the herbs and return to the quartz to your altar.

Spell For Personal Success and Achievement

What you'll need:

- a piece of sunstone

- an orange candle

- pink or kosher salt

- juniper berries

- some soil

- a small bowl, or cauldron

- benzoin incense

- myrrh oil

- small, slim paintbrush

- matches

Cast your circle, and anoint the candle with the myrrh oil. Light the incense. In the bowl or cauldron, place the salt, soil, sunstone, and juniper berries. Mix these with your athame or wand, in a sunwise direction.

As you stir the ingredients, say:

"As the Sun warms the Earth and encourages the harvest,

so does my ability for success grow every day.

I will achieve my goals and dreams, step by step,

as sure as the sunflower and the wheat grows tall."

Picture the sun shining down on a field of wheat and sunflowers: these represent your success and finances. Picture the wind swaying the tall stalks. See how the field spans out endlessly towards the horizon. This is your success, it is tangible and real.

Say:

"As the candle burns its flame, so does my success increase."

When you are ready, open the circle and allow the candle to continue burning down. Sprinkle the spell ingredients except for the sunstone in an open field at your earliest convenience.

Tiger's Eye Self-Esteem Spell

What you'll need:

- a piece of tiger's eye

- a yellow, white, or orange candle

- matches

- a small plate or candleholder

- Solar oil: three drops of rosemary, cedar, and orange oil mixed

- a small, thin paintbrush

Anoint the candle with the solar oil, then light the candle. Stand before it holding the tiger's eye in your hands. Look to the ceiling and imagine the sun. Close your eyes.

Imagine the sun's rays filling the space of your sacred circle. Picture their warmth filling you, soothing every limb, filling you with passion, and with courage. Know that whenever you face a difficult situation, the sun's energy will be there to keep you strong.

Say these words:

"I call upon the energy of the Sun

to imbue this crystal

with your power.

May it be a constant reminder

of my self-worth,

each day I spend

on Earth."

Lift your hand with the crystal and allow the sun to fill the tiger's eye with its bold, confident energy. When you're ready, open the circle and allow the candle to burn down. Keep the tiger's eye in your pocket throughout your days or place it on your altar for daily meditation.

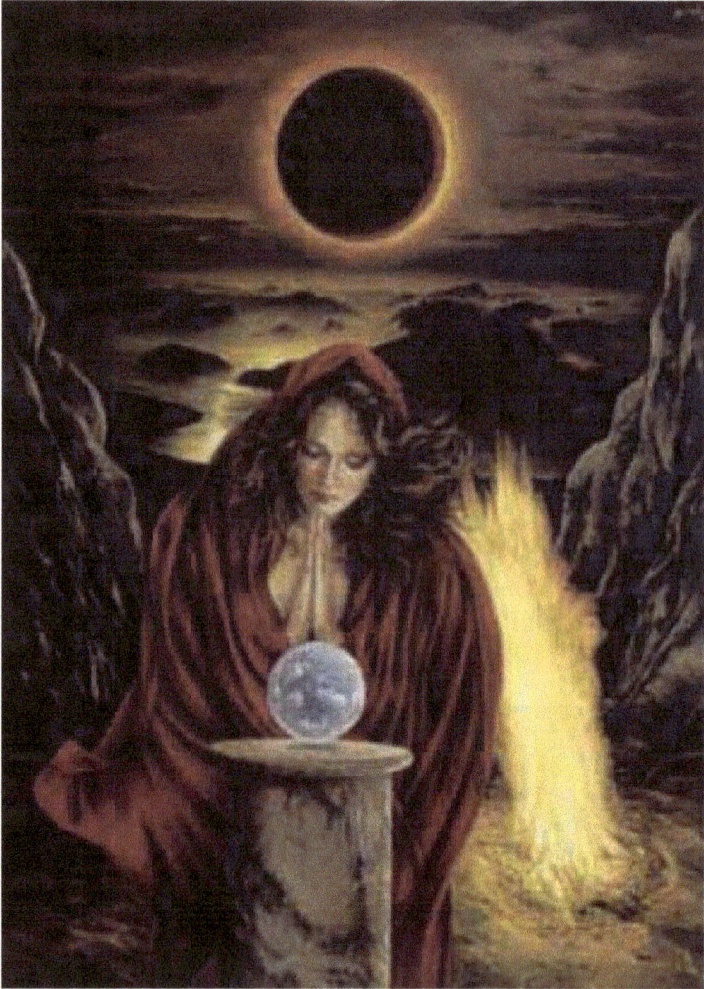

A Spell to Reclaim Power

What you'll need:

- white quarts

- a piece of onyx

- one white and one black candle

- matches

- Sacred oil blend: rosemary, myrrh, frankincense

- a small, thin paintbrush

- Florida water, or holy water

- bundle of sweet grass or hand-picked wildflowers

- a vase or glass half-filled with water

Do this spell on a waning or dark moon. After the circle is cast, anoint both candles and set them on your altar or workspace. Place the onyx and the quartz between them so that from left to right they look like this: black candle, onyx, white quartz, white candle. Take the bundle of wildflowers and lightly sprinkle them with Florida or holy water then shake the water onto yourself using the bundle of wildflowers, from head to toe. Once you've done this, place the wildflowers in the vase on your altar.

Now take the stones and hold them, one in each hand: hold the onyx in your right hand and the white quartz in your left.

Say:

"I take back that which belongs to me,

by the darkness of night and the bright light of day.

I call upon the dark moon's energy,

to guide my thoughts and light the way.

What was stolen is now restored,

and the balance of my mind returned.

By the magic within these stones,

and by the flame of the candle that burns."

Lift your arms, still holding the stones, and feel the energies of your life in perfect balance. Feel your power course through you like the infinity symbol, a figure eight—endless. No one can alter or stop this.

When you are ready, return the stones to their places on the altar, and open the circle.

Simple Spell to Overcome an Obstacle

What you'll need:

- small gathered sticks (you will need at least ten) from the woods: each stick should be approximately 5" long

- dragon's blood incense

- a red candle

- clove oil

- a small, thin paintbrush

- matches

- a candleholder or plate

> Cast the circle, anoint the candle, and light the incense. Take the sticks and one by one, build a small structure. The design is up to you: it can be a little house, a pyramid, or you can stack the sticks five across going one way, five across the other. Make sure the structure is as tall as you can get it.

> While you work on this, describe the obstacle or problem you're wanting to overcome. With each placement of a new stick, describe one facet or fact of the obstacle.

> When you're finished with this work, say:

"By the fiery flame of this candle,

so I ignite my courage."

With one, strong sweep of your hand, knock the structure you've built off of your altar. As you're doing so, imagine your victory in overcoming the obstacle you described.

Say:

"And so it is done."

After you've opened the circle and allowed the candle to burn down, discard the sticks in the woods, a field, or at a crossroads.

Spells For Wealth and Abundance

Changing Your Mind About Money

Before you embark on casting a money spell, take some time to examine your attitude towards money. Unfortunately, many of us have a negative attitude towards money—even if we love getting money and enjoy shopping with it! Those of us who have a *scarcity* mentality are always worried about money running out, and who wouldn't be? Remember that magic is the exercise of will to create change. You can change your financial situation through magic, but you have to stop worrying about money being scarce.

Start changing your outlook today. Every time you spend money, be thankful for it. Actively thank your money for working hard for you—tell it to bring back its friends to you a hundred-fold. Even if you're just paying your phone bill, thank the universe for allowing you to pay it, and thank your money for being there when you needed it.

Bad ways of thinking to get rid of right now:

- I don't deserve to have a lot of money.

- I never make enough money.

- I don't possess the proper education, skills, or talents to make the money I want.

> Remember, never ask "how". The universe knows how— you only have to trust in your strong connection to the universe. If you contradict your magical work, it will fail, plain and simple. You have to change your beliefs first so that your will can create miracles through magic.

> **Practice affirmations.** Anywhere from a full lunar cycle, to a week before you want to cast your money magic spell, take a few minutes each day to repeat a money-related affirmation, such as:

> "I deserve to have the money I desire."

> "I am good at making money."

> "I attract abundance every day."

> "Money is coming to me every day."

Try to stay in the present when you recite affirmations; don't make statements that pertain to the future. Stay in the *now*. And even if you don't yet believe these affirmations, saying them every day will change your thinking, in time. You can choose to light a candle and cast a circle when you recite one or several of these affirmations.

Practice gratitude. When your thinking is gratitude-based, you will stop dwelling on what you lack and start focusing on what you *have*. Take time every day to say out loud or write down something you're thankful for having. BELIEVE what you're saying.

Counter negativity with a question. If you catch yourself slipping back into the old habit of thinking negatively about money, try this exercise. If you find yourself thinking, "I never have enough money," turn it into a question: "Why do I feel as if I never have enough money?" Take time to meditate on the question, let it remain in your thinking as you go about your days. Eventually, you will answer the question subconsciously and the doubt itself will disappear and will no longer rooted in reality. That old, negative belief will no longer haunt you.

Orange Money Spell

What you'll need:

- an orange

- a golden or silver dollar

- a small piece of paper and a pencil

- powdered cinnamon

- basil

- patchouli (herb), or patchouli oil

- orange zest, powdered or crumbled

- vervain

- a brown or green candle

- Abundance oil: a mixture of honey, patchouli oil, lemon oil, and sandalwood

- matches

- a dish on which to burn the candle

- a small, sharp knife

   Perform this spell on a new, waxing, or full moon. Anoint the candle with the abundance oil and light it.

Write on the piece of paper: *money come, money grow, money dance, money flow*. Place the coin onto the middle of the paper and sprinkle the cinnamon, basil, patchouli, orange zest, and vervain onto it.

Fold the paper towards you, then turn it sunwise and fold it once more. Do this as many times as you need to make it small enough to fit inside the orange. Make a small, deep cut in the orange and place the folded spell inside. Place the orange on your altar and keep it there for seven days. After the seventh day, remove the coin and donate it to a charity. Discard the orange and paper.

A Simple Spell For Abundance

What you'll need:

- your cauldron or a silver bowl

- three silver dollars

- collected rain or river water

Perform this spell only on a full moon. Fill the cauldron or bowl halfway with the collected water. As you drop each coin into the water, say:

"Abundance, come to me,

by river, road, air or sea.

I am grateful for this abundance, eternally."

Place the cauldron or bowl where the moon's light can reflect upon the water's surface. The next day, remove the coins and keep them in your pocket, billfold, or purse. Never spend them.

A Treasure Chest

What you'll need:

- a wooden box with a latch

- a coin of every denomination, some foreign coins, and a paper bill of each denomination

- green jade

- pyrite

- clear quartz

- rose quartz

- a bundle of alfalfa, tied with green string

- freshly picked basil leaves

- three bay leaves

- a piece of ginger root

- Abundance oil

- Florida water or orange blossom water

- a spray bottle

- a bundle of sage

- matches

Perform this spell under a full moon. A blue moon (the second full moon in a month) is a particularly good time for this spell.

This is an expensive spell, obviously, but a powerful one. Save it for a time when things are going well, or—save *up* for it to build up your abundance and help keep it going strong. In the spray bottle, mix some Florida or orange blossom water with a few drops of the abundance oil.

Light the sage bundle and gently smudge each coin, bill, and stone. Take the spray bottle and lightly mist each coin, bill, and stone, setting each one inside the box as you do so. As you place each object into the box, say:

"By the power of three times three, this treasure box brings abundance to me."

When you're finished placing all the objects in the box, close the box and place your hand upon it. Say:

"This box is now a magnet for wealth and prosperity

which then flows from this box to me,

that it harm none,

so mote it be."

Set the box in the light of the moon, either outside (where it won't be detected or stolen), or on a windowsill, and say:

"Bella luna,

cast your light

upon this treasure box tonight

and let my magic take flight."

Recharge the box every full moon for continued flow of wealth and abundance. *Note:* if you ever find you're in a situation where you must spend the money in the box, do not worry over it. Use the stones in new ways for continued prosperity, and when you're able, refill and recharge the box.

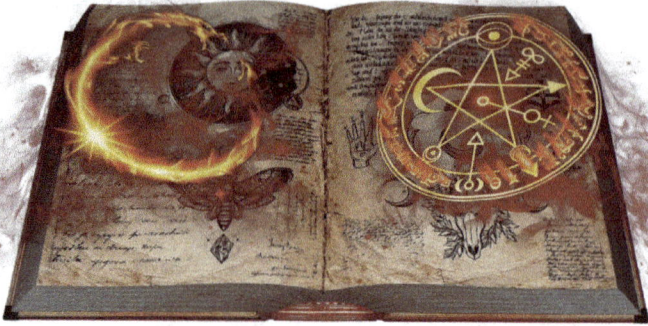

Red Cloth Money Bag

What you'll need:

- a red cloth bag or pouch (small); you can also sew your own

- needle, red thread, scissors if you're using a bag you've sewn yourself

- three golden dollars

- a small mirror—small enough to fit easily into the pouch

- a green candle

- Abundance oil

- a small, thin paintbrush

- matches

- a candleholder or small dish

Do this spell only on a full moon. Anoint the candle and light it. Take time to draw down the power of the moon; holding your hands high, say:

"Bella luna,

come on down,

so lovely, with your silvery crown,

grace this circle with your light

bless my magical work this night."

Feel the powerful, lunar energy coursing down into your circle, filling the space with white light. Drop your hands when you feel the circle is full.

Place the three coins and the mirror into the pouch, then either sew or tie it shut. Hold the bag in your hand while focusing your gaze at the candle's light.

Say:

"Paper and coin,

abundance and wealth,

for joy, for freedom, and in good health,

is mine tonight, and forever on,

beneath the moon's light and the sun's,

to bring me no harm, nor to harm anyone."

Raise the bag up to the moon's light and say: "So mote it be, and so it is done."

After you open the circle, allow the candle to burn down. Carry the bag with you or let it remain on your altar. Additionally, you can place it on top of your wallet when you're at home.

A Simple Candle Money Spell

What you'll need:

- a green candle

- matches

- a dish on which to burn the candle

    Do this spell on the full or waxing moon. Light the candle and very carefully, place your the back of your hand above it, just high enough so that you can feel it warming your hand. Turn your hand in sunwise circles, and say:

    "God and goddess, bring to me $500."

Seven Day Money Money Spell

What you'll need:

- a green candle

- a white candle

- two candleholders or dishes

- Abundance oil or Wealth oil: cedar, frankincense, and rose

- matches

- a small, thin paintbrush

    Do this spell on a waxing or full moon. Anoint both candles and place them approximately seven inches apart from each other and light them. Bring down the power of the moon, raising your arms to the ceiling and saying:

    "Mother goddess, grant me your powerful, lunar energy. Fill this circle with your light."

    Imagine the lunar light filling your circle like rushing water. Drop your arms when the space is full.

    Each time you say the following chant, move the white candle, representing yourself, one step closer to the green candle. Say this chant seven times:

    "Riches and wealth, come to me,

    by the power of three times three,

to bring harm to no one nor to bring harm to me,

Abundance is mine, so mote it be."

Allow the candles to burn for seven minutes, then snuff them out by pinching the flame. Burn them for seven minutes a day, for seven days. On the seventh day allow the candles to continue burning down until they're finished.

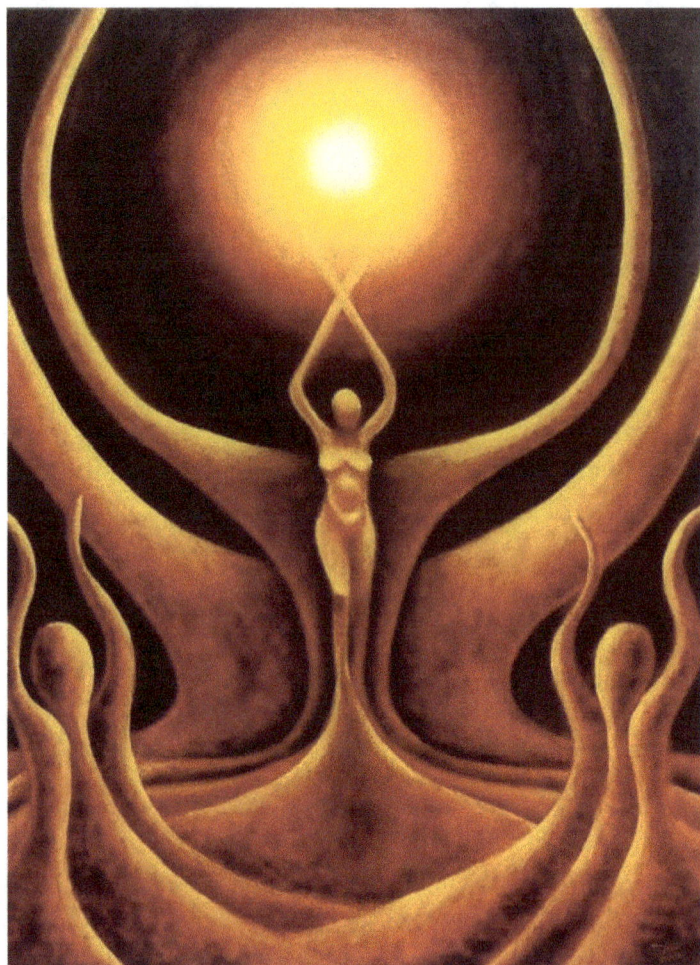

Spells For Love, Happiness, and Relationships

The Heart of the Ocean Love Spell

What you'll need:

- A blue, green, or white bowl

- Seven seashells

- Seven pearls (you can buy a strand of pearls at a craft store—they can be freshwater or saltwater, either is fine for this purpose)

- Ocean sand (easy to find in the floral department of many large stores)

- A blue, green, or white candle

- Matches

- A dish or candleholder

- Pure Love oil: rose, sandalwood, jasmine

- A small, thin paintbrush

- Saltwater (you can make your own with collected rainwater and pink salt, use a teaspoon of salt in this case)

- A piece of green jade, or a moonstone

This is a spell if you believe that you are ready for a healthy, loving, long-term romantic relationship. You are ready to be open to receiving love as well as giving love, unconditionally. Perform this spell on a new, waxing, or full moon. Take time for this spell, do not rush through it. Have a soothing shower or relaxing bath before you begin.

Anoint the candle with the oil and light it. Pour the rainwater into the bowl, and slowly pour in the salt, stirring sunwise as you focus on your open, loving heart. Raise your arms toward the sky and feel the loving, peaceful energy of the moon pour down and fill your sacred circle. Once the energy glows the brightest, let your arms drop. It is time to begin.

Drop the gemstone into the bowl.

Pour the sand into the bowl so that it covers the bottom of the bowl but does not rise above the water. Say:

"Life is change, like the shifting tides.

I am ready for love."

Pick up one of the seashells, imagine yourself filling it with loving patience. Drop it into the water and say:

"Life is a test, and requires patience.

I am ready for love."

Pick up a second seashell. Imagine filling it with laughter and delight. Drop it into the water and say:

"Life is fun, and filled with friendship.

I am ready for love."

Pick up a third seashell, and imagine filling it with peaceful solitude. Drop it into the water and say:

"Life is sometimes a journey alone until we reunite again.

I am ready for love."

Pick up a fourth shell and imagine filling it with passion. Picture embracing your true love, and if you're comfortable, picture kissing them. Drop the shell into the water and say:

"Life will make me hunger for the one I adore the most.

I am ready for love."

Pick up a fifth shell, and imagine filling it with gentle calm. Picture holding hands with your true love, in silence, watching a sunset. Drop the shell into the water and say:

"Life is reflection, together with my equal in life.

I am ready for love."

Pick up a sixth shell, and imagine filling it with strength. Imagine hearing words you do not like, and meeting those darker emotions with a renewed sense of love. Drop the shell into the water and say:

"Life is an occasional struggle, yet I rise to this with even greater love.

I am ready for love."

Pick up the last shell and hold it in your hands clasped. Imagine a lifetime in moving images, happy scenes, scenes of togetherness, scenes of disagreements with loving resolutions, scenes of travel, scenes of accomplishment. Say:

"Life is a winding road that I will walk together with my true love.

I am ready for love."

Drop the last shell into the water. With your hand, or with your wand, trace a sunwise circle above the bowl. Say:

"These ingredients I invest in thee, like all the treasures in the sea, to one day bless us, you and me, together in love, successfully."

Reach into the bowl and remove the stone you dropped in the beginning of the spell. Keep it on your altar or carry it with you as a beacon to your true love that they easily find you in the world. Remember true love takes time. Allow the spell to send its message into the universe, and when the time is right, your true love will appear.

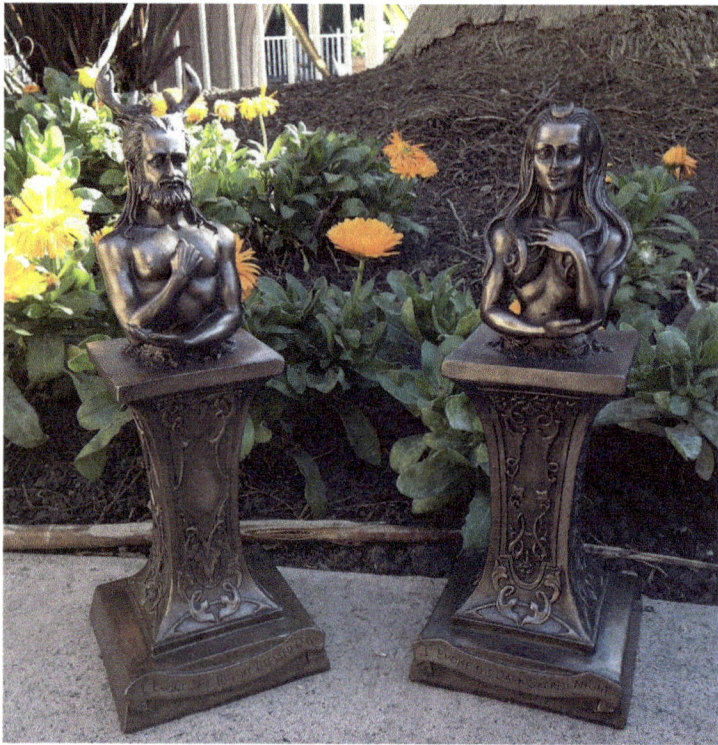

Attracting Love Sachet

What you'll need:

- lavender

- red or pink rose petals

- a cinnamon stick

- rosemary

- yarrow

- calendula

- rue

- lemongrass

- a small piece of paper

- a pencil

- a cloth pouch or bag, in red, orange, purple, or pink, long enough to hold a cinnamon stick

- Red string or yarn

- Three drops of Pure Love oil

In a bowl, mix the ingredients except for the cinnamon stick. On the slip of paper, write this sentence without lifting the pencil (don't worry if it looks sloppy, just do your best): *True Love, come to me.* Tightly roll the paper towards you. Place it against the cinnamon stick, and wrap the string or yarn around it tightly, three times. Say the Casting Words.

Place the herbs in the bowl into the pouch, carefully, then place the cinnamon stick wrapped with the paper. Add three drops of Pure Love oil and tie up the pouch.

Carry the pouch with you, or tie it to your bedpost for one lunar cycle.

A Warm Heart In Winter Spell

What you'll need:

- two pine cones

- red string

- a fireplace or bonfire

    Perform this spell on a waxing or full moon. Tie the pine cones together with the red string, and say "May I be united with my love by the next full moon." Say the Casting Words, then toss the pine cones into the fire to release the spell's energy into the universe.

The Heart's Choice Divination Spell

What you'll need:

- two onions

- two pots and some potting soil

- a small, sharp knife

- collected rainwater

- a pink candle

- a candleholder or a small dish

- matches

- Pure Love oil

- a small, thin paintbrush

> Do this on a new moon. After casting your circle, anoint the candle with the oil and light it. Take the knife and carefully inscribe the name of the two lovers you need guidance about—one in one onion, one in the other. As you carefully plant each onion, say the name of the lover in question.
>
> Put one hand on each pot and call to the goddess:
>
> "Wise and loving goddess, my heart is confused.
>
> Help me know which lover I should choose.
>
> With the first that grows, I will know."

Allow the candle to burn down, and once it has, water the soil well, then place the two pots where they can get the most sun. Whichever onion sprouts first, that is the lover you should choose.

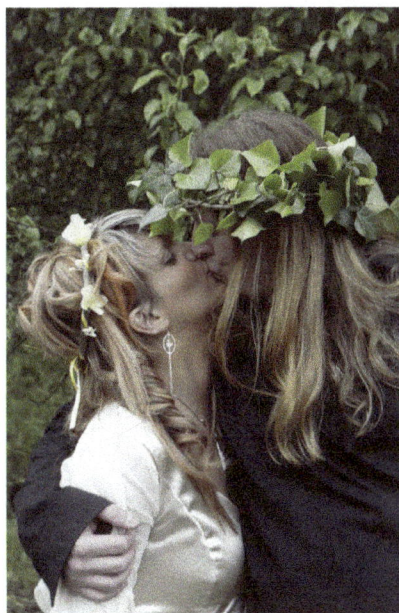

Rose Water Recipe

What you'll need:

- rose petals, enough to fill a mason jar

- collected rain or river water

- cheesecloth

- a pink candle

- Pure Love oil

- a small, thin paintbrush

- matches

- a candleholder or small dish

- pink and white quartz

- a teaspoon of honey

- lemongrass

- honeysuckle blossoms

- one mint leaf

Do this spell on a new or waxing moon and finish it on a full moon. Anoint and light the pink candle. Place the lemongrass, mint leaf, honeysuckle blossoms, white and pink quartz and rose petals into the mason jar then fill to the brim with the collected water. Seal the jar.

Draw down the power of the moon and let it fill your circle as you hold the jar in your hands. Open your eyes when you imagine the moon energy glowing bright.

Say:

"A gentle brew I make for you,

to heal the heart and bring love true."

Imagine the loving energy from your own heart pouring into the jar. Give it three, firm shakes, then set it beside the candle.

Once the moon is visible, place the jar in a windowsill or outside where it can bask in the moon's light. On the night of the full moon, return the jar to your sacred workspace or altar. Say:

"By the light of the goddess moon,

I consecrate this spell to bring

true love soon."

Place it once again in the moonlight. The next day, carefully strain the rose water through a cheesecloth, setting the quartz stones aside to return to your altar for future use. Bottle the rose water to use in future love spells, to sprinkle on yourself before leaving the house if you seek true love, or to give as a gift to a friend who is looking for true love.

A Spell to Strengthen Unconditional Love

What you'll need:

- a black, pink, and white candle

- Sacred Oil blend: myrrh, frankincense, patchouli

- a small, thin paintbrush

- three small dishes or candleholders

- matches

- pink salt

- rose incense

After you cast your circle, anoint all three candles and set the pink candle in between the black and the white candles. Light them, then light the incense.

Draw a figure eight, beginning with the black candle, so that it crosses over the pink candle and encircles the black and white candles. Say:

"Balance divine, yours and mine

neverending, not pretending

strong and true, me and you

in this love, pure and fine."

Set the incense stick to burn in a holder, watch the smoke drift over the candles' flames as you imagine your love strengthening, becoming more balanced and stable. When you are ready, open the circle and allow the candles to burn down.

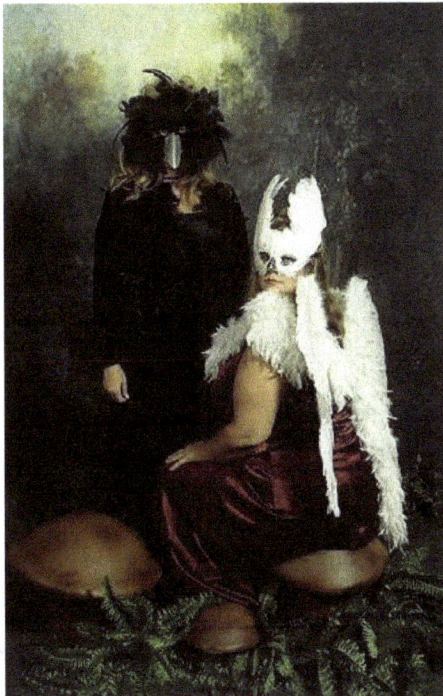

Spells For Healing and Wellness

White Light Healing Spell

What you'll need:

- a wall mirror

- a white pillar candle

- a dish or candleholder

- matches

- five white quartz pieces

You can do this spell at any time. The mirror doesn't have to be particularly large, just big enough that when you set it on the floor, against a wall, you can see your reflection if you're seated in front of it.

Place the mirror against a wall. Place the dish in front of it and set the candle on the dish; light the candle. Sit comfortably in front of the candle. Place the five quartz pieces around you on the floor so that you are surrounded by them. Allow your gaze to shift out of focus and watch your reflection in the mirror bathed in the light of the candle. Take deep, even breaths from your center—your shoulders should not move up and down, your belly should move in and out. Sit with good posture.

See the white, healing light combine with the natural aura of your body. Picture the white light brightening your aura, drawing out any negativity of illness from your body. Feel the healing, cool, white light comfort your body. Watch the new, white aura shimmer and glow. Stay in this state of mind for as long as it's comfortable.

When you are done, extinguish the candle by pinching the flame, and return the mirror to its place. You can do this as a simple meditation, or cast a circle to do it as a magical affirmation.

Calming Waters Spell

What you'll need:

- a blue candle or bouquet of blue or white flowers

  This is a spell that can be done in several places. You can perform it in the bathtub in your home, or in a lake, creek, river, or in the ocean. You don't need any spell ingredients but a candle for focus or a gift of flowers, and yourself, a body of water, and the elementals of water.

If taking a bath, cast a circle and light the candle for divine focus. If bathing in a natural body of water, leave the bouquet of flowers by the shore as thanks to the elementals of water.

This spell should be done on a dark or waning moon. Once submerged in the water, relax, take deep breaths. You can be standing or floating, or if in the bathtub, laying down. Once you've found that your mind is in a calm, healing place, say these words:

"Elementals of water, guardians of the rain

Elementals of water, fair spirits of the stream,

Elementals of water, children of Yemaya,

Elementals of water, shepherds of the sea,

Help me release all the worry, the stress,

the negative thoughts that trouble me.

Here in your safe, calming currents, I swim peacefully."

Feel the gentle embrace of the water, the push and pull of currents if you are in a natural body of water. Feel the cool, healing of the goddess and her elementals, surrounding you, comforting you, healing your pains, and worries. Remember that the goddess can handle all of the pain you release to her, she is infinite. Allow the stress to be taken from you. You are a child of the goddess, and she is a loving mother to all her children.

Take some of the water and wet the top of your head with it, thus anointing yourself. Feel the coolness of the water refresh your third eye and your crown chakra.

When you are ready, leave the water and allow the air to dry you, or pat yourself dry—do not wipe the healing water away.

Healing Candle Spell

What you'll need:

- a blue, white, or yellow candle

- Healing Oil: angelica, comfrey, and chamomile

- a small, thin paintbrush

- a dish or candleholder

- matches

- Tibetan healing incense

- an incense holder

- a small knife, or screw

Cast your circle and anoint the candle. With the small knife or screw tip, carve the words "heal me" in both sides of the candle, then light the candle. Light the incense and allow the smoke to drift across the candle flame, filling the room with a healing scent. (Place the incense far enough away from you so that you are not directly breathing the line of smoke). Allow your mind to drift into an alpha state: your gaze is out of focus, your mind is calm, thoughts are discarded as they enter the space of your mind. As the candle burns, know that you are in the right place for healing of the spirit, mind, body, and soul. Feel the benevolent energy fill your circle. Feel the power of the universe filling your circle with healing light.

When you are ready, open the circle and ground. Allow the candle and incense to burn down.

Earth Cord Spell

This spell is a simple but powerfully effective one. On a full moon, find space to work unbothered and unobserved out of doors. Stand barefoot if you can but if the weather is cold or the ground too rough, shoes are fine.

Cast the circle around you and look up to the sky. Call the power of the sun or the moon into your circle, silently or out loud, and feel the energy of the universe slowly fill your sacred space until the space is completely filled with divine power.

Stand straight, with good posture, and breathe deeply, keeping your arms relaxed at your sides. Imagine a silver cord of energy going from your solar plexus, to your belly, down through your feet and deep into the Earth. Feel the exchange of energy from your body to the body of the goddess. With each breath, feel the healing coming up from the ground into your body.

At the same time, feel the negativity, stress, weariness, and worry leave your body through the silver cord, to be carried down into the Earth where it will be dissipated and cleansed, and renewed as bright, healing energy. Stay in this stance for as long as you need, allowing the goddess to heal your body, heart, and spirit.

Burying a Bad Habit Healing Spell

What you'll need:

- an egg

- a brown candle

- Tibetan healing incense

- Healing Oil

- a small, thin paintbrush

- a small dish or candleholder

- a shovel

- a brown paper bag

- a pencil

On a dark or waning moon, prepare your body first by bathing or showering. Cast your circle, and anoint the candle with Healing Oil. Light the candle as well as the Tibetan healing incense. Raise your hands to the sky and ask the god and goddess to grace your sacred circle with their healing energy. Imagine the circle filling with divine energy, and open your eyes when the energy glows the brightest.

Write on the paper bag the habit you wish to get rid of; be specific and detailed. Next, take the egg, and say:

"Little egg, a vehicle be

to remove the habit which vexes me,

so that I may see that habit undone

by the rise and set of the burning sun."

Now, take the egg, and slowly and gently rub it against you (careful not to break it!), starting with the top of your head, down to your face and neck, your shoulders and arms, your chest, ribs, and stomach, your lower back and buttocks, each leg and ankle, down to your feet and out over your toes. Place the egg carefully in the brown paper bag, and fold the bag so that it forms a small package. Move this package carefully and slowly, widdershins (counterclockwise), above the candle, careful not to get so close that the bag begins to burn. Say the Casting Words.

Open the circle and allow the candle and the incense to burn down while you go outside with the parcel and a shovel. Dig a small hole and bury the egg in the paper bag, and forget about it. In 24 hours' time, your bad habit should begin to dissipate, until it vanishes forever.

Sunrise Affirmation Spell

Perform this spell on a waxing, new, or full moon. Research at what time the sun will rise at your location. Make sure you get plenty of sleep the night before this spell. Set your alarm to wake you up with enough time to shower, drink some water, and feel refreshed and ready.

Stand facing East, preferably outdoors, but in front of an east-facing window is also permitted. As the sun rises, say:

"Like the sun,

each day I rise,

I will not stop,

nor compromise.

With each breathe,

I live and grow,

I will not stop,

onward, I go."

Feel the energy of the rising sun imbue you with strength, hope, and vitality. Make a commitment to do a sunrise affirmation once a month. The sunrise is a magical time, and being awake during it can be very healing for anyone, but especially those in the creative or healing arts. The dawn is a great source of inspiration, and of hope.

Spells For The Home and Garden

House Blessings Jar

What you'll need:

- a mason jar

- collected water such as rainwater or water from a river

- amethyst, white quartz, jade, and sunstone

- vervain

- comfrey

- rosemary

- alfalfa

- juniper berries

- any wildflowers that are growing on the property, such as dandelions

- honey

- some soil from outside the property, or the nearest park if the home is an apartment

- a coin of each denomination, including a silver dollar

- sage, palo santo, rosemary, or holy water (collected water and salt)

- sweet incense

- a yellow or green candle

- matches

Perform this spell on a new, waxing, or full moon. Especially powerful when performed on a blue moon (a second full moon in a month). Cast your circle around the entire home: if this is a house, you can walk around the outside of the house, or walk from room to room going north, east, south, then west.

Next, purge any negativity from the rooms using sage, palo santo wood, rosemary, or holy water. The holy water should be sprinkled in each room, walking widdershins about each room, all other ingredients should be lit so they smoke, and by holding them, making widdershins hand motions with the smoke in each room.

When you are finished cleansing the house, open the windows and doors, keeping an eye on small children and pets.

After a few minutes, close the windows and doors, and walk the house with the sweet incense, making sunwise hand movements to bless each room.

Finally, return to your altar and begin assembling the jar. Add the ingredients: soil and stones first, then coins, honey (save a little bit of the honey to anoint the candle), herbs, wildflowers, and last, water. Seal the jar.

Melt the bottom of the candle to affix it to the lid of the mason jar. Anoint the candle with the remaining honey, then light the candle.

Say:

"Bless this house,

this cozy home,

a place of peace,

back home to come,

let good luck grow

and bless these rooms,

let happiness flow,

often and soon,

peace to this home,

and who dwell within,

where love and light,

come pouring in,

by day and night,

through thick and thin,

this house is blessed,

and all within."

Allow the candle to burn down, and open the circle. Light another candle on the jar whenever you wish to reactivate it, on a full or new moon, reciting the words.

House Cleansing Ritual

What you'll need:

- a household broom or magic besom

- Florida or holy water

- kosher salt and pepper

On a dark or waxing moon, and after securing all pets and small children, open the exterior doors of your house. Sprinkle Florida water or holy water lightly on the floor in front of you, and sweep it towards the doors, beginning in the center of the house. You can put the water in a spray bottle to lightly mist the floors, especially if there is carpet. Do this in each room until you're in the rooms that lead to the outside, and continue sweeping until you reach the thresholds. Sprinkle a small amount of salt and pepper on the thresholds, then sweep the water, salt and pepper outside, taking with it all the negative energy that's been tracked in.

Take care to thoroughly sweep the salt and pepper so nobody tracks it back in, and pets don't carry it on their paws. Another approach is to sew small cloth packets of salt and pepper mixture and place these on the thresholds to ceremoniously collect the negative energy to sweep out of the house.

Garden Blessing Spell

What you'll need:

- white quartz flakes

  Do this spell on a new, waxing, or full moon. It is best done in the morning or in the evening, whenever your garden is in shade and when you typically water your plants. At your altar, set a pitcher of water and light a white candle. Cast your circle and call down the energies of the sun and the moon, and ask them to fill the water with their healing light. Open the circle and carry your pitcher out to the garden, bringing with you a pocket of quartz flakes. Water your plants as you would, then take each flake and set it a couple of inches into the soil among your plants, pouring the blessed water on top of it as you work. When you are finished, say:

  "With blessings of the moon and sun,

  my garden grows, one by one."

Spells For Protection

Front Door Protection Charm

What you'll need:

- a clove of garlic

- red cloth bag

- three needles or pins

- rosemary

- sage

- Crown of Success oil or Dragon's Blood oil

- African violet petals

- twine

- scissors

On a Tuesday or Saturday of a dark or waning moon, cast your circle and press the pins carefully through the clove of garlic. Carefully place the garlic into the cloth bag, and add to this the rosemary, sage, garlic, African violet petals, and six drops of oil. Close the bag and wrap it three times in twine, making a loop from which you can hang the bag on or near the front door.

Hold the bag towards the moon, and say:

"From this moment, from this hour,

trouble keep far from my door,

I use my cunning and my power,

to keep that which would harm me far away, forevermore."

Say the Casting Words. Affix the bag to the front door, or close to it. Recharge it twice a year with six additional drops of oil, and repeat the incantation.

Witch's Jar

What you'll need:

- a mason jar or any household food jar that once held something sour, such as pickles, or sauerkraut

- a collection of rusted, metal objects: screws, nails, hooks, etc.

- broken glass (not mirrors)

- vinegar

- a lock of your own hair, and some of your fingernail clippings

- a black candle

- matches

- a candleholder or small plate

A witch's jar performs a simple function. Interestingly, it was once believed that one could trap a witch within such a jar—today, however, the witch's jar is a way to trap negativity, ill will, and animosity that's directed towards you.

On a dark or waning moon, light the black candle and place everything from the list inside the jar. Seal the jar and drip some of the wax from the candle on the lid, and say:

"All that serves to harm me, come inside this jar and stay."

Snuff out the candle and take the jar outside to bury it. Some witches make four jars in total, one for each side of the house. If you rent or live in an apartment or any home without a yard, you can place the witch's jar in a pot of gardening soil. You can even place a live plant in the pot— perfect camouflage for your jar!

Four Corners House Protection Spell

What you'll need:

- four black cloth bags

- four small, circular mirrors

- twine

- kosher salt

- black peppercorns

Remember that black is an important color in protection magic and should not be considered "evil" or "dark". Just as the darkness of night protects animals who need protection against predators so do we sometimes use the color black to keep us hidden from our enemies.

Cast a circle on a dark or waning moon. Place inside each cloth bag a mirror, a pinch of kosher salt and a pinch of black peppercorns. Tie up the bags and bind them each three times with twine, making a loop in one of the binds so the bag can be hung, if you choose. Hold each bag in your hand and say for each one:

"Invisible to misfortune,

my home remains a safe haven.

Invisible to trouble,

my home remains safe,

behind a black wing, like the raven."

Place one bag on each side of your house. You can hang it from a window or place it on the ground, whichever you prefer.

Invisible From Harm Personal Protection Spell

What you'll need:

- a fresh basil leaf

- a dime

- a piece of onyx

- white yarn, or any thick, white thread.

- Crown of Success oil

- a small, sharp knife or boline

- a black candle

- a white candle

- two candleholders or two small dishes

- matches

On a dark, new, or waning moon, cast your circle. Carefully carve the words "Trouble do not see me" on each candle. Place the candles on your altar, one candle to each side of you, and the ingredients in the middle. Take the basil leaf and place the dime upon it, then the piece of onyx upon that. Carefully wrap the three items together with the yarn or thread, concentrating on being able to walk about in the world, free from harm, not troubled by others. When you are finished, tie three knots while you say:

"Trouble do not see me." Say the Casting Words.

Carry this charm in your pocket, backpack, briefcase or purse to keep harm from finding you.

Safe Journeys Spell

What you'll need:

- a white rose (only the flower, removes the stem)

- a white feather

- a white cloth bag

- a lodestone

- nag champa incense

- matches

A lodestone can be purchased in a pagan supplies shop or online. Do this spell during any lunar phase but the dark moon. After you cast your circle, light the incense. Hold the white rose blossom and circle it sunwise with the incense, then place it in the bag. Do the same for the white feather, and for the lodestone. Tie up the bag and hold it up, then circle it three more times with the incense. Say:

"May this blessed charm, filled with light,

bring safe travels, day and night."

You can make this charm for a loved one or friend who's planning on traveling, or for yourself before a trip. You can also keep it in your car to keep you safe while you drive on daily errands or your commute.

As with all charms, you can recharge this one under a full moon when you feel the need to.

Invisible Ward Spell

What you'll need:

- kosher salt

- collected water, such as rainwater or river water.

- obsidian

- a black candle

- Crown of Success oil

- a small, thin paintbrush

- a small glass, or your cauldron or cup

- a small knife or your boline

  Do this spell under a dark moon. After you cast the circle, carve a figure eight symbol in the black candle, and anoint it with the Crown of Success oil. Fill the container you've chosen to use with the collected water, then add a teaspoon of salt. Take the piece of obsidian, and make a figure eight symbol in the air directly above the container of water.

  Say:

  "Infinity circles, day and night,

  charge this water

  to keep me out of sight."

Drop the obsidian into the water. Place the cup outside or in the windowsill to soak up the dark moon's energy. Allow the candle to burn down.

Keep the invisibility water in a bottle or spill-proof container. When you want to use it, either paint a small figure eight on your body (good places are your chest or stomach, anywhere where the salt residue won't be seen), or on your front door, or vehicle, depending upon the context of your need for invisibility.

Spells For Luck

Birthday Blessings Spell

What you'll need:

- a tall white pillar or taper candle

- a small, sharp knife or your boline

- Altar oil: frankincense, rose, lemongrass

- Florida water

- a small, thin paintbrush

- a small dish or candleholder

- matches

Do this spell on your birthday, regardless of lunar phase. If it occurs on a waning moon, be prepared for unnecessary or harmful things to begin to move out of your life, so that the happiness can move in.

Cast your circle and carefully carve two-word wishes into the candle, such as: "gentle love", "happy home", or "satisfying work". Use your imagination and carve what you truly want for the coming year. Anoint the candle with the altar oil. Light the candle. Take the Florida water and place a small amount on the top of your head, your forehead, the back of your neck, and on the back of your hands.

Gaze at the candle's flame, and imagine scenes in which the things you've carved occur, or could occur. Take deep, calming breaths from your stomach, and sit with a straight posture. Take some time in this sacred space, breathing, and meditating on the happy year you have in front of you. Even if you've recently suffered a trauma or loss, imagine the year bringing you healing, and solace from the pain.

When you are ready, open the circle and ground, but allow the candle to burn down on its own.

Nutmeg Spell

What you'll need:

- a whole nutmeg

- frankincense oil

- a dollar bill

- red string or yarn

Do this spell on a full moon. Cast your circle, and hold the nutmeg in your hand as you call upon the energy of the moon to fill your sacred spice with lunar energy. Dab a bit of frankincense oil on the nutmeg, then wrap it in the dollar bill. Next, bind the wrapped nutmeg in red string, seven times. Tie the knot three times, and say:

"Lucky charm, bold and bright,

bring me luck both day and night."

Allow the charm to bask in the light of the full moon, then carry it on your person, bag, car, or altar.

Seven Berries Spell

What you'll need:

- seven juniper berries

- a small green or white bag

    Begin this spell on a Sunday during a waxing moon—
    making sure that the full moon is at least seven days away.
    Cast your circle and place the juniper berries in the bag.
    Hold it in your hands and allow the power of the sun and
    the moon to fill your circle, and charge the berries.

    Carry the berries on you for seven days. After that, discard
    them in running water. You will then have a very lucky
    week.

Help With Legal Issues Spell

What you'll need:

- red jasper

- hematite

- small white cloth bag

- High John the Conqueror root

- Success oil: basil, myrrh, dragon's blood, rosemary

- small, thin paintbrush

- the Justice tarot card

- the World tarot card

- the Empress tarot card

- a small, yellow candle

- matches

- a candleholder or small dish

- a red apple

Do this spell on a waxing or full moon, on a Monday or a Friday. Before you begin, thoroughly cleanse yourself both physically and spiritually. Smudge your altar space and tools.

Anoint the candle and light it. Allow its warm glow to soothe your anxiety about the upcoming court case or legal issue.

Take the High John root, which can be purchased online or in a magical supply store, and consecrate it with the success oil. Hold it to your forehead and say:

"Justice be gentle, and favor me,

Empress be loving, and comfort me,

World be open for me to journey,

may things go my way, successfully."

Place the High John root in the bag. Stand the three cards up behind the candle or on the altar so you can gaze at them. Take the red jasper in your left hand, the hematite in your right, and look at the cards, one at a time, as you repeat:

"Justice be gentle, and favor me,

Empress be loving, and comfort me,

World be open for me to journey,

may things go my way, successfully."

Place the jasper and hematite in the bag and tie it securely. Now take the Justice card and place it on top of the bag. Say:

"Justice, find all in favor of me that I will be successful in my endeavors." Return that card to the altar.

Take the Empress card and place it on top of the bag. Say:

"Empress, mother goddess, soothe my fears and let those who I deal with have mercy on me." Return that card to the altar.

Take the World card and place it on top of the bag. Say:

"Universe, enable it so that I keep my liberty and dignity, and am allowed to walk my path uninhibited in this World." Return that card to the altar.

When you are finished, allow the candle to burn down. Take the remaining wax and the apple and place in a crossroads at your earliest convenience.

Conclusion

Thank for making it through to the end of *Wicca Spells*. Let's hope it was informative and able to provide you with all of the tools you need to achieve your goals whatever they may be. Through this book, you learned a bit on the origin and history of Wicca, its beliefs and practices, some of the tools used by Wiccans, the elements and the Wheel of the Year, and how to perform spells. Among the spells included in this book are those that attract luck in wealth, money, love, as well as protection of home and safe travels.

The next step is to begin to research what you want out of magic. Do you want to change your life? If so, how? Start with small details and see if one area of your life needs more attention than the rest. Once you've decided what aspect you'd like to focus your first spell upon, start to look up the phases of the moon, the times of sunrise and sunset where you live, and which days of the week would be best to perform this spell. See what ingredients are needed, and go about collecting them. Take your time, and enjoy the process of preparing to cast your first spell.

Once you're ready to create magic, remember to relax and have fun with it. A mistake is not a dealbreaker—whatever you do, do so with good, strong intent, and you will see the results better than you imagined.

You may instead choose to pick a spell in this book and just go for it. That's okay too! Curiosity in magic leads to miraculous things. Learning keeps us alive and filled with the energy of the god and goddess. So, test the waters, explore, be brave—and know that every spell in this book has been crafted with the new witch in mind.

Finally, if you want to go slow and gradually build your altar, gather and purchase your tools, grow a magical herb garden, and wait until the time is right for you to delve into the world of Wiccan magic, that is okay, too. There is no wrong way to honor yourself in Wicca. Choose the path that's right for you.

Finally, if you found this book useful in any way, a review on Amazon is always appreciated!

CPSIA information can be obtained
at www.ICGtesting.com
Printed in the USA
BVHW092051190421
605311BV00002B/117

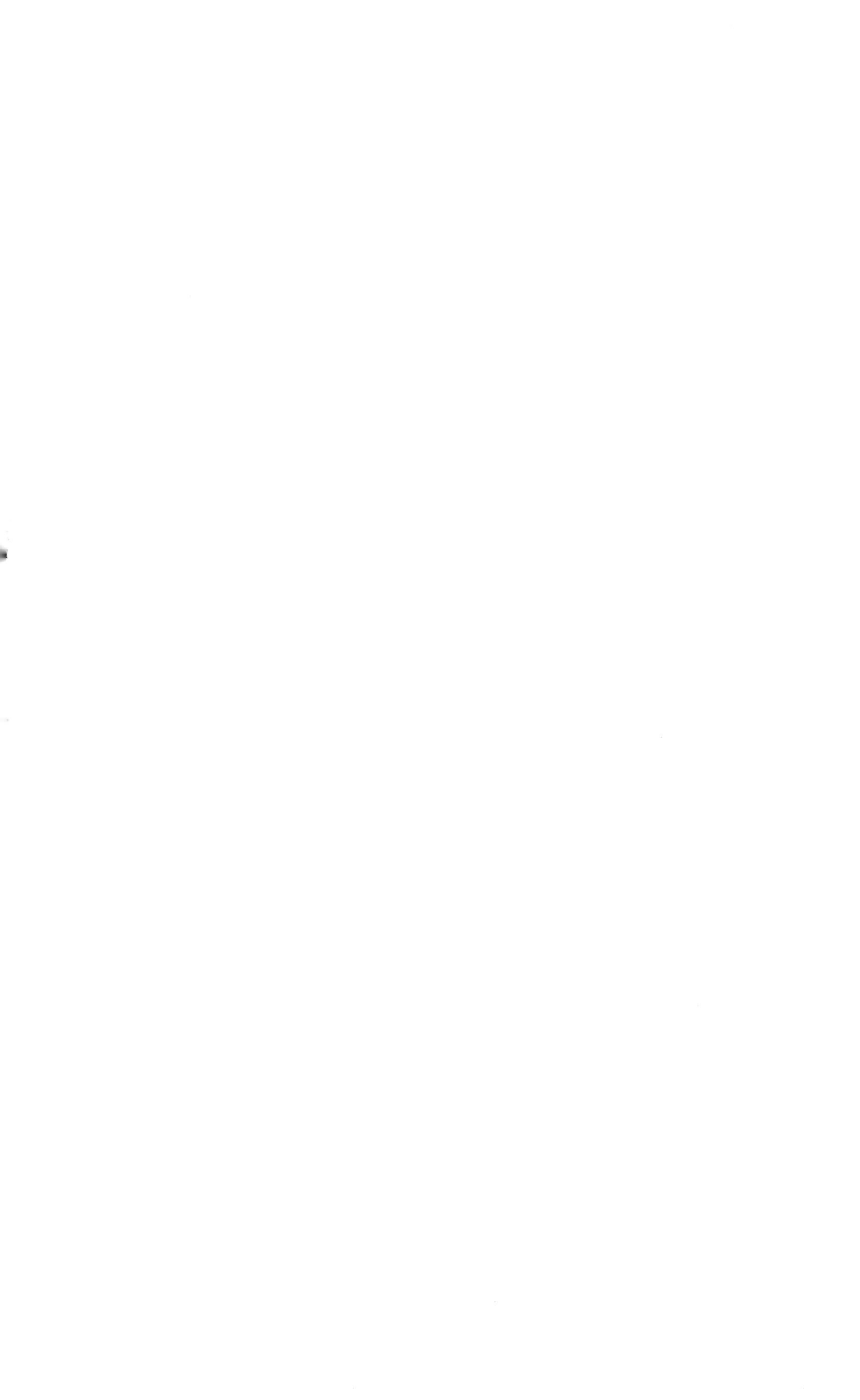